14 Days of Clean Eating for Lasting Li.

14 Days of Clean Eating for Lasting Lifestyle Change

The content of this book is for general instruction only. Each person's physical, emotional and spiritual condition is unique. The instruction in this book is not intended to replace or interrupt the reader's relationship with a physician or other professional. Please consult your doctor for matters pertaining to your specific health and diet.

To contact the publisher or author, visit:

www.cherylbohonyi.com

ISBN 978-0997518801

Printed in the United States of America

14 Days of Clean Eating for Lasting Lifestyle Change

14 Days of Clean Eating

Sometimes we need a little kick-start, a short period of time where we are really strict with what we eat so we can feel better immediately! That's exactly what you're getting here, along with some great lifestyle habits to carry with you after your 14 days.

I don't like the term "detox diet" since it implies that your body can't function and remove toxins as it is designed to do. As long as your organs are all functioning properly and you don't have any medical conditions, there is no reason to detox or cleanse. This is more like a "spring cleaning" meal plan, as it removes many of the foods we tend to overeat and have really negative effects on our body and our mood!

Are you scared yet? Don't be! Let me tell you a bit about the results people have gotten by following this plan for 2 short weeks:

Rachel says: "Down 9.2 pounds and 7 inches overall. Woohoo! Best challenge out there! Nutritional mindset has changed and I am so excited for this new lifestyle! First 3 days were tough, but once you commit, it's so worth it!"

Kathi says: "Amazing program with great results! 8 pounds lost! The first few days may be tough, but it's definitely worth it! A wonderful lifestyle change that is easy to carry with you once the challenge is over. You won't want to go back to your old habits."

Sandy says: "I know it's not about the scale, but I had not lost all my "baby weight" and it's been 7 years. I have tried everything and this has finally worked for me. This is the best plan I have ever had and I have not felt this good in years!"

Are you convinced to give it a try? On the next few pages, you will get some general guidelines about clean eating. Then you will see a complete meal plan and recipes for 14 days along with a shopping list. You just choose one of the options for each of 3 meals and 2 snacks every day. Follow the plan and watch your body, energy and mindset transform!

What is clean eating?

Clean eating can have many definitions, depending on who you ask. One thing that is universal, though and is the heart of clean eating is eating whole foods, as close to their natural form as possible, with minimal processing. Vegetables, especially leafy greens should make up about 50% of your diet. Sounds like a lot right? Think about how many servings of vegetables you are currently eating in a day. Not even close? That's EXACTLY why you need a plan like this!

Second comes protein, most of which should be plant based. Everything you eat has protein in it, so it is highly unlikely that you aren't eating enough. The best plant-based sources of protein are nuts and seeds, leafy greens, broccoli and whole grains. Quinoa is a complete protein that can be used in place of rice in any recipe. For animal proteins, I recommend including whole eggs, fish and chicken or turkey. Beef, pork, lamb, venison and other meats should only be included occasionally.

Getting plenty of healthy fat in your diet is the key to feeling satiated and dramatically reducing cravings! Great sources include fish, such as salmon, nuts and seeds, avocado and whole eggs.

Lastly, I highly recommend choosing organic products as much as possible. This will limit your exposure to pesticides and fertilizers and generally provide you with a better quality food.

As for fruit, most of us are eating too many servings in a day! Yes, fruit is good for you and has a nice array of vitamins, fiber and antioxidants, however, you only need 2-3 servings per day to get that nice array. A serving of fruit is a small apple or banana or a cup of berries or grapes. Remember, fruit still has sugar, even though it is natural sugar, and too much is still too much! Have a serving with breakfast and a serving for a morning snack or lunch.

Starting with these steps eliminates falling back on carbohydrates to fill up on. We tend to fill up on low quality carbs, like bread, cookies, cakes, chips, pretzels and crackers. When you start by filling half of your plate with vegetables, you aren't hungry for these processed foods that weigh you down and sap your energy!

Eat leafy greens every day!

Yes, I will mention this again, as so many of us aren't getting enough of these nutritional powerhouses in our diet! There are so many leafy greens available now, so there's no reason to get bored eating the same thing all the time. Also, by having them daily, I don't mean you have to eat a salad every day. That is a quick and easy way to get it in, but there are plenty of other tasty ways to do it too!

Eat a variety of greens each week, rather than eating the same thing every day! Romaine, iceberg and butter lettuces are okay, but try some of the dark leafy greens too: kale, collards, swiss chard, spring greens, broccoli greens, arugula, even the greens from carrots and beets! Get creative – for example, one of the suggested meals in the 14 day plan has you using collard greens as a wrap for sandwiches. Other suggestions in this meal plan include using leafy greens at breakfast, with your eggs, and in smoothies. Don't limit yourself based on what you disliked growing up. Your tasted buds have changed! Go ahead and give some of these different varieties a try!

Do not skip meals!

One of the worst things we do to ourselves is skip meals. Skipping breakfast sets you up for major cravings all day. Many people I talk to will slug down a cup of coffee as soon as they get up in the morning, then they aren't hungry for breakfast. Well, it's time to stop that! A good breakfast sets your metabolism for the day and helps get your body ready, energetically, for the day.

Are you a lunch skipper? Why? Do you think you're too busy to stop for a mid-day meal? Schedule a lunch time for yourself. Again, you're not doing yourself any favors by skipping it.

How about eating at your desk? Is this you? It's time to stop that too! Take notice of the executive management at your place of work. Are they eating at their desk? My guess is probably not! Yes, you can take 20-30 minutes for lunch. Actually, taking that time away from your desk will help energize you and make your more productive all afternoon! Go ahead and take a quick walk outside after you eat too, if you can. You'll immediately notice a difference in your mood and will be much more productive all afternoon.

Snacks

During this 14 days, it is important to include a morning snack and an afternoon snack. As you go through it, you may eliminate the morning snack, simply because there is usually only a few hours between breakfast and lunch. An afternoon snack, however will keep you from getting too hungry by dinner time and ultimately overeating as a result.

Reduce your carbs

We've already talked about carbohydrates a bit, but I wanted to dive in to it and get a little more specific. At least 75% of your carbohydrate intake should be in the form of vegetables! You can eat any kind of veggies you like without too much restriction, but definitely be careful of what you add to it. Use herbs and spices to change up the flavors but limit how much butter and oil you use. While butter and (olive, coconut) oil are fine to use, you want to be aware of how much you use and keep it to a minimum.

The other 25% of your carbohydrates can come in the form of fruits and whole grains. Whole grains do not include whole grain breads, pasta and other processed carbs. Whole grains include brown rice, quinoa, millet, amaranth, kasha, oats, farro, teff, etc. See one on the list you've never had? Give it a try!

Let's talk about quinoa

Quinoa is technically a seed, although it is used as and often referred to as a grain. Quinoa is very versatile. Not only can you use it in place of rice, but you can also use it in place of oats for a breakfast option. Breakfast is actually my favorite way to enjoy it – with a dab of butter, cinnamon and strawberries.

Prepare a large batch of quinoa once per week and use it all week in all kinds of meals – breakfast, cold in salads, in stir fry. There are no limits! I prefer to buy it in bulk and typically cook it in water so it doesn't absorb any other flavors and I can use it in any application. It also tastes great cooked in chicken or vegetable broth, but that limits your use of that batch.

Simple cooking directions: 2 cups quinoa, rinsed (very important!) with 4 cups water. Bring to a boil, then simmer, covered, for 12-15 minutes until all the water is absorbed and you can see the spirals.

Plan ahead!

Planning is the key to success! If you don't plan, you will fall into the "what's for dinner" trap. As demonstrated with the quinoa, you can prepare some things in advance for use throughout the week. For this plan, I've done much of the planning for you, but you need to do the prep work! Nothing in this plan is complicated to make and, when you prepare in advance, most of the meals can be put together in just a few minutes.

Here are some great meal planning tips to use after the 14 days, adapted from my meal planning workshop:

- Set aside an hour to focus on planning your meals for the first time.
- Write out the days of the week on a piece of paper and create columns for breakfast, lunch, dinner and snacks.
- Once you've got your meals all planned out, write your shopping list. Pull out recipes and review them to be sure you get everything you need!
- Plan to spend a little time prepping some of your food after you shop.
- Don't be afraid to experiment with new recipes, but try them on days when you have more time. Don't try to reinvent the wheel when you have to run out the door!
- Keep breakfast simple (i.e. scrambled eggs with spinach and/or sweet potatoes or oatmeal with fruit) on mornings when you have to get out quick. Have just one or two breakfast options all week.

- Prep what you can in advance. When chopping veggies for a dish, chop extra, leave some raw and cook some extra (exceptions: tomatoes, potatoes). Boil a dozen eggs at a time and store them in a clearly marked egg carton (in their shell).
- Packing lunches can be easy! Again, have just a couple of choices each week. Hard boiled eggs are a good start and you can add some raw veggies and maybe a slice of gluten free bread with hummus or guacamole for dipping. Have to eat out? Go for broth based soups without noodles, salad with grilled chicken or grilled chicken or fish and vegetable platter. Always ask for your meat grilled rather than sautéed (often dredged in flour) or breaded.
- Don't stress out about dinner time! Make sure everyone has their afternoon snack so dinner can be light and relaxed. Some great snacks include fruit with nuts or nut butters (peanut butter, almond butter or cashew butter), a smoothie made with frozen berries, spinach and almond milk, veggies with hummus or guacamole, or a hard-boiled egg with grape tomatoes.
- If you only shop once a week (really, who has time to go more?), plan to shop on the weekend, then stop at the farm market/CSA or have a delivery of fresh fruits and veggies mid-week.

Drink water!

Make water your primary (or only) beverage. You can throw some fruits or veggies and herbs into it if you need a boost of flavor. Some great choices are lemon, berries, cucumber, other citrus fruits, mint, pomegranate, etc. Use a combination that sounds good to you!

During your 14 days, you should not consume anything other than water (that includes coffee!). Many people balk at that, but it really makes a big difference in your energy level and how you feel overall. To help avoid coffee cravings, try having warm lemon water in the morning. Yes, you will probably have a headache for the first day or two, but I promise, you'll feel so much better by eliminating the coffee! So, again, no coffee, tea, juice, soda, not even sparkling water.

Let's talk about alcohol. Surely you've read something to justify your daily wine or beer habit. Well, I'm here to tell you to step away from the drink! Having 7 drinks in a week dramatically increases your risk of alcohol dependency and increases your risk of cancer, especially breast cancer up to 150%! Ignore those claims that a glass of wine before bed will make you lose weight or that beer is the best recovery drink after a run – they're simply not true!

Ditch Gluten and Cow Dairy

I know what you're thinking – another restriction that makes this plan impossible. Well, just hear me out and see how you feel then.

Gluten can be very difficult for people to digest and many people have a sensitivity to it and don't even realize it! Also, gluten is sneaky and shows up in products you wouldn't think it would – like salad dressing! This is about more than having a sandwich! Going gluten free is a trend for a reason. Gluten tends to cause bloating and discomfort, as well as contribute to skin issues, brain fog, energy drain and more. Does that mean you'll never have bread again? No! What it means is that you will go gluten free for these two weeks, then re-introduce it slowly to see how it actually makes you feel.

Similarly, we will forgo cow dairy. It isn't the products themselves, but the casein in cow dairy that gives us a hard time. Give goat milk products a try, even sheep milk cheeses and buffalo mozzarella are okay to include. Substitute almond, rice or coconut milk where you would use cow's milk. All of these items are easier to digest and don't typically cause the bloating that cow dairy often does.

So, here's the plan:

- Follow this meal plan for 14 days. Pick from one of the 3 choices for each meal. You'll have breakfast, morning snack, lunch afternoon snack and dinner. You won't have anything to eat between dinner and breakfast.
- Time your meals so that you are eating ever 3-4 hours. For example, if you get up at 5 in the morning, have your breakfast by 6, morning snack around 9, lunch around noon, afternoon snack around 3 and dinner around 6.
- Drink plenty of water throughout the day.
- Enjoy your meals!

Meal choices (Fall and Winter)

Breakfast

> ➢ 2 scrambled eggs with sautéed spinach or kale
>
> ➢ ½ cup (before cooking) plain oatmeal (instant is fine, just make sure there's no added sugar), made with water with ½ cup berries
>
> ➢ Green smoothie – go light on the fruit! Skip the sweeteners!

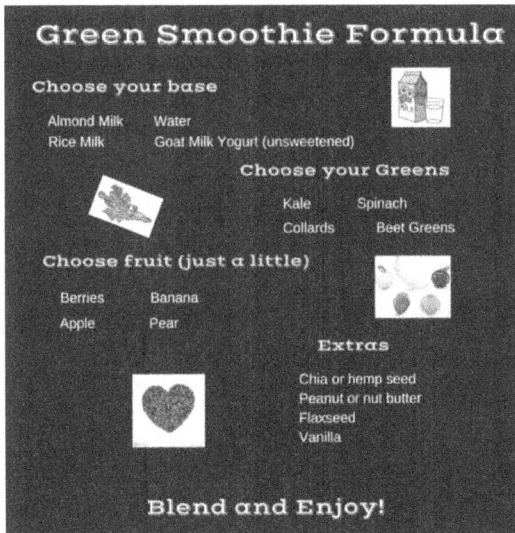

Green Smoothie Formula

Choose your base

Almond Milk   Water
Rice Milk   Goat Milk Yogurt (unsweetened)

Choose your Greens

Kale   Spinach
Collards   Beet Greens

Choose fruit (just a little)

Berries   Banana
Apple   Pear

Extras

Chia or hemp seed
Peanut or nut butter
Flaxseed
Vanilla

Blend and Enjoy!

Morning Snack

> ➤ Small apple with 1 Tablespoon Almond or Peanut butter (with no added sugar)
> ➤ Small banana with ¼ cup walnuts
> ➤ ½ cup berries mixed into 1 cup plain goat milk yogurt

Lunch

> ➤ Mixed greens with variety of veggies (tomatoes, peppers, corn, cucumber, zucchini, etc.) with oil and vinegar dressing (use extra virgin olive oil and any vinegar you like – balsamic, red wine, white wine, apple cider, etc.) If you like some crunch, add sunflower seeds, pumpkin seeds, almonds, walnuts or other nuts.
> ➤ Chicken salad
> ➤ Make a wrap using collard greens

Afternoon Snack

> ➤ 5 baby carrots with 1 Tablespoon hummus
> ➤ 1 hard-boiled egg with 2 celery stalks (sprinkle with sea salt)
> ➤ ¼ cup trail mix (make your own using any combination of nuts and seeds). For sweetness, add coconut flakes, but skip the dried fruit

Dinner

- ➤ Shredded chicken with salt and pepper (hot or cold) with green beans, asparagus, broccoli or a small salad
- ➤ Fish (salmon, tuna, striped bass, flounder) with mixed veggies, baked sweet potato
- ➤ Buffalo chicken salad

Week 1 (Fall and Winter)

Day	Breakfast	AM snack	Lunch	PM snack	Dinner
Day 1	Smoothie	Apple	Salad	Carrots	Chicken & veggies
Day 2	Eggs	Banana	Chicken salad	HB egg	Fish
Day 3	Oatmeal	Yogurt	Wrap	Trail mix	Buffalo chicken salad
Day 4	Eggs	Apple	Salad	HB egg	Chicken & veggies
Day 5	Oatmeal	Banana	Wrap	Trail mix	Fish
Day 6	Smoothie	Yogurt	Chicken salad	Carrots	Buffalo chicken salad
Day 7	Eggs	Apple	Wrap	HB egg	Chicken & veggies

Week 2 (Fall and Winter)

Day	Breakfast	AM snack	Lunch	PM snack	Dinner
Day 8	Oatmeal	Banana	Salad	Carrots	Fish
Day 9	Smoothie	Yogurt	Wrap	Trail mix	Buffalo chicken salad
Day 10	Eggs	Apple	Chicken salad	HB Egg	Chicken & veggies
Day 11	Oatmeal	Banana	Salad	Trail mix	Fish
Day 12	Eggs	Yogurt	Chicken salad	Carrots	Buffalo chicken salad
Day 13	Smoothie	Apple	Wrap	Trail mix	Chicken & veggies
Day 14	Eggs	Banana	salad	HB egg	Fish

Meal choices (Spring)

Breakfast

➢ 2 scrambled eggs with sautéed spinach or kale
➢ ½ cup (before cooking) plain oatmeal (instant is fine, just make sure there's no added sugar), made with water with ½ cup blueberries
➢ Green smoothie – go light on the fruit! Skip the sweeteners!

Green Smoothie Formula

Choose your base

| Almond Milk | Water |
| Rice Milk | Goat Milk Yogurt (unsweetened) |

Choose your Greens

| Kale | Spinach |
| Collards | Beet Greens |

Choose fruit (just a little)

| Berries | Banana |
| Apple | Pear |

Extras

Chia or hemp seed
Peanut or nut butter
Flaxseed
Vanilla

Blend and Enjoy!

Morning Snack

- ½ cup strawberries with 1 Tablespoon Almond or Peanut butter (with no added sugar)
- Small banana with ¼ walnuts
- Raspberries w/sunflower seeds

Lunch

- Mixed greens with variety of veggies (tomatoes, peppers, corn, cucumber, zucchini, etc.) with oil and vinegar dressing (use extra virgin olive oil and any vinegar you like – balsamic, red wine, white wine, apple cider, etc.) If you like some crunch, add sunflower seeds, pumpkin seeds, almonds, walnuts or other nuts.
- Chicken salad
- Make a wrap using collard greens

Afternoon Snack

- 5 baby carrots with 1 Tablespoon hummus
- 1 hard-boiled egg with 2 celery stalks (sprinkle with sea salt)
- ¼ cup trail mix (make your own using any combination of nuts and seeds). For sweetness, add coconut flakes, but skip the dried fruit

Dinner

- ➢ Shredded chicken with salt and pepper and any other spices you enjoy (hot or cold) with green beans, asparagus, spring peas or a small salad
- ➢ Fish (salmon, tuna, striped bass, flounder) with mixed spring veggies
- ➢ Spring vegetable soup

Week 1 (Spring)

Day	Breakfast	AM snack	Lunch	PM snack	Dinner
Day 1	Smoothie	Strawberries	Salad	Carrots	Chicken & veggies
Day 2	Eggs	Banana	Chicken salad	HB egg	Fish
Day 3	Oatmeal	Raspberries	Wrap	Trail mix	Spring veggie soup
Day 4	Eggs	Strawberries	Salad	HB egg	Chicken & veggies
Day 5	Oatmeal	Banana	Wrap	Trail mix	Fish
Day 6	Smoothie	Raspberries	Chicken salad	Carrots	Spring veggie soup
Day 7	Eggs	Strawberries	Wrap	HB egg	Chicken & veggies

Week 2 (Spring)

Day	Breakfast	AM snack	Lunch	PM snack	Dinner
Day 8	Oatmeal	Banana	Salad	Carrots	Fish
Day 9	Smoothie	Raspberries	Wrap	Trail mix	Spring veggie soup
Day 10	Eggs	Strawberries	Chicken salad	HB Egg	Chicken & veggies
Day 11	Oatmeal	Banana	Salad	Trail mix	Fish
Day 12	Eggs	Raspberries	Chicken salad	Carrots	Spring veggie soup
Day 13	Smoothie	Strawberries	Wrap	Trail mix	Chicken & veggies
Day 14	Eggs	Banana	salad	HB egg	Fish

Meal choices (Summer)

Breakfast

- ➢ 2 scrambled eggs with sautéed spinach or kale
- ➢ ½ cup (before cooking) plain oatmeal (instant is fine, just make sure there's no added sugar), made with water with ½ cup berries
- ➢ Green smoothie – go light on the fruit! Skip the sweeteners!

Green Smoothie Formula

Choose your base
Almond Milk   Water
Rice Milk   Goat Milk Yogurt (unsweetened)

Choose your Greens
Kale   Spinach
Collards   Beet Greens

Choose fruit (just a little)
Berries   Banana
Apple   Pear

Extras
Chia or hemp seed
Peanut or nut butter
Flaxseed
Vanilla

Blend and Enjoy!

Morning Snack

- Small apple with 1 Tablespoon Almond or Peanut butter (with no added sugar)
- Small banana with ¼ walnuts
- ½ cup berries mixed into 1 cup plain goat milk yogurt

Lunch

- Mixed greens with variety of veggies (tomatoes, peppers, corn, cucumber, zucchini, etc.) with oil and vinegar dressing (use extra virgin olive oil and any vinegar you like – balsamic, red wine, white wine, apple cider, etc.) If you like some crunch, add sunflower seeds, pumpkin seeds, almonds, walnuts or other nuts.
- Chicken salad
- Make a wrap using collard greens

Afternoon Snack

- 5 baby carrots with 1 Tablespoon hummus
- 1 hard-boiled egg with 2 celery stalks (sprinkle with sea salt)
- ¼ cup trail mix (make your own using any combination of nuts and seeds). For sweetness, add coconut flakes, but skip the dried fruit

Dinner

- ➢ Shredded chicken with salt and pepper (hot or cold) with green beans, asparagus, broccoli or a small salad
- ➢ Fish (salmon, tuna, striped bass, flounder) with mixed veggies, baked sweet potato
- ➢ Buffalo chicken salad

Week 1 (Summer)

Day	Breakfast	AM snack	Lunch	PM snack	Dinner
Day 1	Smoothie	Strawberries	Salad	Veggies	Chicken & veggies
Day 2	Eggs	Watermelon	Chicken salad	HB egg	Fish
Day 3	Oatmeal	Raspberries	Wrap	Trail mix	Vegetti
Day 4	Eggs	Strawberries	Salad	HB egg	Chicken & veggies
Day 5	Oatmeal	Watermelon	Wrap	Trail mix	Fish
Day 6	Smoothie	Raspberries	Chicken salad	Veggies	Vegetti
Day 7	Eggs	Strawberries	Wrap	HB egg	Chicken & veggies

Week 2 (Summer)

Day	Breakfast	AM snack	Lunch	PM snack	Dinner
Day 8	Oatmeal	Watermelon	Salad	Veggies	Fish
Day 9	Smoothie	Raspberries	Wrap	Trail mix	Vegetti
Day 10	Eggs	Strawberries	Chicken salad	HB Egg	Chicken & veggies
Day 11	Oatmeal	Watermelon	Salad	Trail mix	Fish
Day 12	Eggs	Raspberries	Chicken salad	Veggies	Vegetti
Day 13	Smoothie	Strawberries	Wrap	Trail mix	Chicken & veggies
Day 14	Eggs	Watermelon	salad	HB egg	Fish

Recipes

If you are using lemons for your water, buy organic, slice and freeze wedges.

More on smoothies: use 1 cup base, a nice handful of greens, 1 small piece of fruit (or ½ cup berries), then add any additional protein you might like. I don't recommend protein powders – go for the nut butter, chia seeds or even rolled oats. Cinnamon or other spices are great additions, but skip adding any sweetener.

Once per week, throw skinless, boneless chicken breast into the crock pot (no seasoning, no liquid) and cook on low for 5-7 hours until tender. Shred it with a fork and store in a container in the fridge. Voila! Now you can use it all week long!

Chicken Salad– using ½ cup shredded chicken, mix with shredded carrots, chopped celery, and onion if you like. Combine with ½ smashed avocado. Add slivered almonds if you like some added crunch. Can be eaten as is or stuffed into ½ of a cucumber, sliced lengthwise with seeds scooped out, rolled in a lettuce leaf or stuffed in the other half of the avocado.

Collard wraps– fill with ¼ cup shredded chicken, veggies (peppers, onions, tomatoes, carrots, celery, lettuce, etc), then wrap up just like you would with a tortilla

Suggested way to prepare your green beans, asparagus or broccoli, heat a sauté pan over medium heat. Add just enough vegetable broth to barely cover bottom of pan; when broth is simmering, add your veggies, cover and steam for 5 minutes (3 for asparagus). Remove from heat, add sea salt and enjoy!

Grilling fish - Make foil packets with fish (except salmon), veggies, olive oil, salt and pepper. Close the packets up and put on grill for about 10-12 minutes until fish is cooked through. You can also wrap your sweet potatoes and place them on the grill for about 15 minutes. Salmon can be plank grilled for best flavor. If it's too cold to grill, this same process works in the oven, but it will take a bit longer to cook through – cook at 375-400.

Buffalo Chicken Salad– toss ¼ cup shredded chicken with hot sauce (not wing sauce!) and heat through. Place on a bed of mixed greens, add cucumber, tomatoes, peppers (hot if you can handle it!), corn, etc. No dressing necessary! If you aren't a fan of buffalo sauce, skip the sauce and use an oil and vinegar dressing instead.

Spring Veggie Soup

2 Tbsp olive oil; 2 medium carrots, diced; 1 leek, trimmed and diced; 1 celery stalk, diced; ½ tsp each salt and pepper; 2 cloves garlic, minced; 5 cups veggie stock; 1 cup (fresh or frozen)green peas; 1 cup asparagus, cut into pieces; 2 cups fresh baby spinach; 1 tsp fresh thyme; ¼ cup fresh basil

Heat large saucepan over medium heat. Add oil to coat bottom. Add carrots, leek and celery. Cook about 5 minutes, stirring occasionally; add salt, pepper and garlic. Cook 1 minute, stirring frequently. Add stock, bring to a simmer over medium-high heat. Reduce heat to medium, add peas and asparagus; simmer 4 minutes. Add spinach, thyme and basil; cook 1 minute. Ladle into bowls and enjoy!

Variation: you can use chicken stock and add some cooked, shredded chicken with the spinach step to make a heartier soup.

Vegetti with fresh cold tomato "sauce"

Using a spirilizer (available at most stores or on Amazon for $10-30), make vegetti using zucchini, carrots, cucumber or any other firm veggie or combination of veggies you like.

For the "sauce" – chop tomato, cucumber and sweet peppers into bite size pieces. Add salt and pepper, white wine vinegar and a drizzle of olive oil and let marinate while you create your vegetti. Serve over your spirilized veggies.

Shopping List (Fall and Winter)

Per week – will feed 4 people

2 pounds boneless, skinless chicken breast
4-8 fish fillets (each piece should be about the size of your hand, including fingers)
1 bunch kale
1 bunch spinach (or 1 bag of baby spinach)
Collard greens
2 bags mixed greens – try getting 2 different blends each week
Tomatoes, peppers, cucumbers, zucchini, etc. (whatever your favorites are)
Carrots (buy organic pre-shredded to save some time)
Organic baby carrots
Celery
Green beans
Broccoli
Asparagus
Sweet potatoes
Berries (your favorite ones or any combination)
4-6 small bananas
4-6 small apples
Lemons, if you need them for your water
Almond or peanut butter (small jar or 3-4 individual pouches)
Variety of nuts and seeds (try buying from the bulk bins to save money!)

Plain oats (instant packets are fine as long as they don't have any added sugar)
Olive oil and vinegars, if you don't already have on hand
2 dozen eggs
1 container plain hummus
Plain goat milk yogurt
Almond milk or coconut milk, if you will be making smoothies

Shopping List (Spring)

Per week – will feed 4 people

2 pounds boneless, skinless chicken breast
4-8 fish fillets (each piece should be about the size of your hand, including fingers
1 bunch kale
1 bunch spinach (or 1 bag of baby spinach)
Collard greens
2 bags mixed greens – try getting 2 different blends each week
Tomatoes, peppers, cucumbers, zucchini, etc. (whatever your favorites are)
Carrots (buy organic pre-shredded to save some time)
Organic baby carrots
Celery
Green beans
Asparagus
Blueberries
Raspberries
Strawberries
4-6 small bananas
Lemons, if you need them for your water
Vegetable stock
Almond or peanut butter (small jar or 3-4 individual pouches)
Variety of nuts and seeds (try buying from the bulk bins to save money!)

Plain oats (instant packets are fine as long as they don't have any added sugar)
Olive oil and vinegars, if you don't already have on hand
2 dozen eggs
1 container plain hummus
Plain goat milk yogurt
Almond milk or coconut milk, if you will be making smoothies

Shopping List (Summer)

Per week – will feed 4 people

2 pounds boneless, skinless chicken breast
8 fish fillets (each piece should be about the size of your hand, including fingers
1 bunch kale
1 bunch spinach (or 1 bag of baby spinach)
Collard greens
2 bags mixed greens – try getting 2 different blends each week
Tomatoes, peppers, cucumbers, zucchini, etc. (whatever your favorites are)
Green beans
Asparagus
Blueberries
Raspberries
Strawberries
Watermelon
Lemons, if you need them for your water
Almond or peanut butter (small jar or 3-4 individual pouches)
Variety of nuts and seeds (try buying from the bulk bins to save money!)
Plain oats (instant packets are fine as long as they don't have any added sugar)
Olive oil and vinegars, if you don't already have on hand
2 dozen eggs

1 container plain hummus
Almond milk or coconut milk, if you will be making
smoothies

Congratulations on completing the 14 Day challenge! After making such great progress in a short time, I don't want you just go back to what you were doing before! Here are some tips to easing into your new routine without gaining back what you lost!

- ✓ Keep up with eating 3 meals and 2 snacks per day. Eat your last meal before 7 pm and don't eat anything after dinner.
- ✓ If you're going to reintroduce coffee, make it black, no sugar. And have just 1 cup per day, ideally 2 hours after you wake up.
- ✓ Consider green tea instead of coffee – still with no sugar, 2 hours after you get up.
- ✓ Limit alcohol to 2 drinks per week. Remember all alcohol is sugar!
- ✓ Save sugary items for special occasions – no need to indulge daily!
- ✓ Keep limiting processed foods! Introduce more whole foods, especially veggies!
- ✓ Keep fruit to 2-3 servings per day. (remember a serving is one small piece of fruit or 1 cup of berries, grapes).
- ✓ Watch your portions!
- ✓ Limit red meat to once per week – this includes beef, lamb, pork and wild game.
- ✓ If you choose to reintroduce gluten, do it slowly – once per week. Note how you feel after you have it, whether it's bread, pasta or

even a tortilla – sometimes gluten can make you feel really tired and/or bloated.

✓ If you choose to reintroduce cow dairy, get the best quality you can find – organic, grass fed, whole milk; real butter; real cream or half and half (not fat free), full fat cheeses, full fat, no sugar (or sugar substitute) yogurt, etc. Again, note how you feel. If you don't feel good after you have it, then don't eat it! Try buffalo mozzarella and goat or sheep milk cheeses, as they are easier on your digestive system.

✓ Enjoy your food! No matter what you're eating, the more you enjoy it, the less you need to feel satisfied!

As a final note, remember that caffeine and sugar are highly addictive and neither serves your body well! Use them sparingly. You're feeling good now, so do you really want to go back to how you felt before?

14 Days of Clean Eating for Lasting Lifestyle Change

www.ingramcontent.com/pod-product-compliance
Lightning Source LLC
Chambersburg PA
CBHW071436200326

41520CB00014B/3716